The Gym Life

50 Ways To Lose Weight

50 Sure-Fire Ways To Lose Weight and Burn Fat Without Wasting Time, Money, Or Your Life In The Gym

By Colin Stuckert
AGymLife.com

Contents

Welcome To A Better You

Welcome to a better you. Yes, you... and only you... are responsible for making your training, your fitness and your life, better.

How are you going to do this? Simple...

You are going to take action.

You can read every fitness book, article, or forum in the world and you might ooze with more fitness advice than you can possible contain, but what does that do for you if you don't put in work?

It does this: <u>nothing</u>.

Knowledge is power.... yes, I firmly believe this, but that's not it...

Knowledge is power *if applied*.

If you read this book and learn a bunch of useful tips that can improve your fitness but do nothing about it, then you have squandered your time and money, and I'm not fulfilled as a writer. Don't do that, please, for both of us.

I want you to read and act. Then, when you leave a review on Amazon (thank you, btw), it'll be easy to leave a positive one because you'll refer to the results you got from the action you took. You'll get results, be a happy customer and I'll have accomplished my mission for writing this in the first place. See, we both win.

Let's both win. OK? Good, I'm glad you agree... now get to it!

Yours in Fitness,

-Colin Stuckert

P.S. Make sure you download all the free GymLife guides over at www.GymLifeClub.com. You'll also get my weekly email every Sunday where I share exclusive motivational pieces reserved only for my list.

P.P.S. If you have any questions or comments, email me. I'm here to help. (Ismynamecolin@gmail.com)

It's A Lifestyle

The first 20 ways to lose weight in this book represent the most important aspects of developing health and fitness. If you become proficient in 1 through 20, you will bring your health and performance to the upper levels of your genetic ability. Basically, you'll become the best you can be. I recommend you focus on 1-20 until they are hammered into habit. After that, you can start adding the other tips to your program in small doses to help you overcome plateaus and take your results to new levels.

Keep in mind that these aren't fly-by-night efforts that you can do once or twice and expect results. The recommendations in this book are based on the assumption that you will put in consistent work for long periods of time. If you want lasting results from the 50 tips you are about to read, you will have to build habits around them. Habits are the foundation. They allow you to stay consistent without having to expend willpower (which is a depleting resource) to maintain them. This should be your primary goal in all of your health and fitness pursuits: *to build habits*.

Without further ado, let's get to it!

50 Ways To Lose Weight

1. Eat a grain-free, gluten-free diet of Real Food

The diet that follows these guidelines is called a Paleo, Primal, Caveman, or Hunter Gatherer diet. No matter what you call it, or what variation you decide to pursue, the key is based on one thing: **eating real food**. Real food is food that is pure and raw and that has been unaltered by man. This is what Homo sapiens are made to eat.

Just as gorillas and horses have a diet natural to their species, so do humans. The natural human diet consists of food found in nature. For example, it was not easy to find sugar in the wild. Thus, we are not meant to eat it with any kind of regularity (yet we do, and it's the leading cause of obesity). We are made to eat seafood and animals as a healthy portion (pun intended) of our diet, with vegetables, fruits, nuts and seeds filling in the gaps. The thing is, most people don't need to worry about the quantity of food because they have much more pressing matters to attend to like the **quality** of the food they are eating. When you are eating fast food, frozen dinners, and other cheap, processed food, the only thing that you need to worry about is changing that to real food. After you get the real food habit down, you can start tweaking the amounts of carbs, protein and fat to support your specific goals.

The most important, potent, and best recommendation I can give you will always be: **Eat Real Food**. These three little words represent the cure to obesity and could put an end to factory farming and the fake-food corporatism that monopolizes our food supply and the health of our country.

As humans, we are all held to the same set of rules dictated by the living organism that is currently holding our head and heart. No matter how hard you or I try, we cannot escape our biology. The most important rule of your human body is you must eat real food.

Ignore this rule and you kill yourself.

If you make it your focus to only eat food that is real, you won't have to read books or articles or measure your food with a scale. You don't have to understand science or nutrition. You'll also look better naked, improve your blood markers, and ward of cancer, heart disease, auto-immune disorders and the plethora of other things that eating crappy food uses to kill you.

Real food pretty much fixes everything. And it's so simple— *just eat real food.* I can give no better advice for losing weight, body fat, getting toned, getting stronger, avoiding disease, being happier, and regulating your hormones—and all while promoting health and longevity.

Nutrition is a huge subject that is beyond the scope of this book. Check out the following authors for more information: Robb Wolf, Mark Sisson, and aGymLife.com (yours truly).

2. Get Lots And Lots Of Sleep (And Lots)

I have a love-hate relationship with sleep. I love feeling rested and full of energy, but I hate sleep because it's going to consume—and already has—a third of my life. That sucks. What I realized, though, is I want the other two-thirds of my life to be as awesome as possible, and to make that happen I have to get my 8 hours every night.

The number of hours you need might be different than what I need. You have to figure out what works for you. That said, just because you can operate well on your current schedule does not mean that it is sufficient. Some of you have been sleep deprived for years. As a general rule, 8 hours is the gold standard, but you'll still have to figure that out for yourself.

Start sleeping in a bit more here and there and gauge how you feel. If you start feeling you "need" sleep the more you get it, it's likely you are sleep-deprived. To figure out your "nightly" number, you should first get caught up on your sleep debt. For a couple weeks, start sleeping in a bit more. As you start sleeping more, you'll start getting a feel for what you need to feel good during the day. The more you hone in on this number, the better. When you think you are caught up, try waking without an alarm clock. Then take note of how many hours you get each night. Your average will be somewhere around there.

Once you figure out your average, make sure you go to bed at least that amount of time from when you have to wake up. Make that number your nightly sleep goal.

If you are struggling with weight loss, sleep could be the silver bullet for busting through your plateau. I've seen clients struggle with the last stubborn 5 or 10 pounds for months before implementing more sleep, and like clockwork, they always shed the weight.

3. Practice Intermittent Fasting (IF)

There are many misconceptions surrounding fasting, one of which is that there is only one way to do it. The fact is there are many ways you can implement fasting into your program, and everyone should have some form of fasting built into their eating program. Like eating real food, there is quite a bit of research that suggests we are made to eat sporadically and with long hours between meals. Without going into a full thesis on why you should fast, I will tell you that you should at least be reducing how often you eat as a general weight-loss and health goal. Don't buy into the "multiple small meals" hype meant to sell bars and protein supplements. Six meals a day to "rev" your metabolism is nonsense. To learn more about the benefits of fasting, I highly recommend you check out these resources: MarksDailyApple.com and Leangains.com.

This is the fasting protocol I follow:

Wake: Eat nothing and make Bulletproof Coffee.
4–6 hours later: Train first or eat first meal (depending on schedule)
6-7 hours after first meal: Eat second/last meal of the day (dinner).

My daily fasting goal is to consume my calories within an 8-hour "feeding window." By compressing the time I eat to only 8 hours per day, I end up with a 16-hour fast that starts after my last meal and ends with the next day's breakfast (which, for me, is sometime around 4-5pm). The easiest way to implement this is to base the feeding window on the first meal. As long as I make sure my last meal always comes within 8 hours of "breaking the fast," I'm good until the next day. (For those of you who are not aware, 'breakfast' means to 'break the fast.' It does not mean 'eat first thing in the morning.' Your first meal, whenever that is, is your breakfast.)

While this is my preferred method of fasting, there are other methods you can try. I suggest you experiment and figure out what works for you. Some people prefer to fast by skipping food an entire day once or twice a week. Others try to increase the time between their daily meals. Some prefer to eat one large meal a day and others prefer two or three (I do two a day).

Fasting key points:

1. Fasting does not mean calorie restriction (but it can help you limit calories if that's your goal).
2. The main factor in fasting is meal timing—how frequently you eat.
3. The premise of fasting is the longer you go between eating, the more you grant your body the benefits of hormone regulation, appetite control, increased insulin sensitivity, and much more.

Give fasting a try; it can change your life!

Another benefit of fasting is it simplifies your eating. You are no longer a slave to the "I'm hungry" feeling that dictates so much of most people's lives. When you regulate your hormones, you don't suffer from the nagging blood sugar issues that frequent eaters do (which is most people). This allows you to decide when you want to eat instead of your body calling the shots. It's a better way to live in more ways than one.

Fasting could be your gateway to a whole new set of life-changing results. I highly recommend giving it a try.

4. Eat Slow and Chew Your Food

One way to minimize fat gain during mealtime is to slow down how fast you eat by spending more time chewing your food. This does two things. First, by eating slow, you are controlling how fast calories enter your bloodstream, and thus, spike your hormones—namely insulin. Insulin is a storage hormone, meaning it tells your body to store calories in fat cells. The more insulin you "spike" in your body, the more likely you are to convert those freshly eaten calories into unwanted fat cells. (This is another reason why drinking calories—even protein shakes—is not ideal for weight/fat loss.) By slowing the rate that food enters your blood stream, you are limiting the amount of damage insulin can do. You are, in effect, *regulating your hormones.*

Another benefit of chewing and eating slow is the digestion process. Digestion is a high-energy process that can make you feel sluggish and tired. The more partially chewed food you swallow, the more your body has to expend extra energy to process that food in your stomach, and this slows you down big time.

Your teeth—and saliva enzymes—are designed to break down the tough animal proteins and cellulose walls in plants so your body can better digest and get access to the nutrition inside. Humans have many tools to aid in digestion: fire (cooking food), chewing, stomach acid, and saliva enzymes. Animals that live on predominantly plants, like horses and gorillas, spend the majority of their waking hours chewing food. How often do you see cows or horses not grazing? The point here is chewing is fundamental to the process of digestion for humans, and by rushing it, you are throwing a wrench in the system. The act of mastication (chewing) has also been proven to release extra stomach acid to aid in the process—cool, huh?

By spending more time chewing, you are giving your body the best means of digesting your food while also preventing the large insulin spike that comes with eating food too fast.

Another benefit of chewing and eating slow is you give your stomach time to release the "I'm full" hormone that signals to your brain that you are satiated. We all know what happens when we eat too fast: we get that sickly "full" feeling. This is what happens when you don't give your body enough time to "realize" it's full. No bueno.

Eating slow takes practice. Consider setting a timer to time your bites or start putting your fork down between each bite— or both.

5. Cook Your Food At Home

Let's think about the restaurant business for a moment. Are you picturing your favorite food joint in your head? What do you see as the <u>main</u> difference between your favorite grub-spot and your kitchen at home? It's this:

<u>The restaurant must turn a profit!</u>

Because restaurants are forced to turn a profit, management will do everything they can to reduce costs and raise revenue. It's business 101. Well, do you know where a large chunk of these cost-saving initiatives take place?

The food!

Not only are restaurants doing everything they can to save on food costs by using cheap ingredients, preservatives, pre-packaged sauces, and so on, but they are also trying to make their food taste good and be as addictive as possible. This translates to more refined sugar, salt, MSG, and flavorings that keep you addicted and coming back for more.

For 99.99% of restaurants, your health is not a consideration—or it's only a consideration after the numbers make sense (and even then, they usually use labeling tricks to make you think the food is 'healthy').

When you cook at home, you control the food you eat. As far as eating goes, this is the only way you can have full control of your health. Restaurant food (sans a very few exceptions) <u>is simply not good for you</u>.

Restaurants use cheap oils like soybean, safflower, sunflower, and canola oil to fry cheap ingredients full of gluten, grains, and other preservatives. They reuse fry oil over and over with more of it breaking down with each use. They use sauces that are made in factories halfway around the world. Their produce is sprayed and shipped from who knows where. And don't get me started on how unsanitary restaurant kitchens are; the kitchens are in the back, and out of sight, for a reason. Think about it.

All in all, it's time you got in the kitchen and started preparing your food from fresh ingredients. Grab my book: The Gym Life Book of Cooking Technique (GymLifeCook.com) for a crash course in teaching you how to cook meals without a recipe by learning basic techniques you can use over and over.

6. Go Gluten-Free

I won't go into the many reasons why you should be eating gluten-free because I don't have room here. (Check out MarksDailyApple.com for further reading on the benefits of going gluten-free.)

In simple terms, humans aren't made to eat grains, especially processed, refined ones. Humans develop various autoimmune and gut disorders from eating grains and the lectins in them.

To figure out if grains are causing you a problem (hint: they are), cut them out of your diet for 30-60 days and see where your results go. Then, when you see the results firsthand, you'll never go back.

7. Don't Drink Calories

When you drink calories, you cause a larger than normal insulin spike due to the speed the calories enter your blood stream (like eating fast). We are not made to drink calories. In nature there are very few liquids that contain calories (milk was not a standard part of our ancestors' diet until after agriculture became widespread, and even then it wasn't pastured or homogenized).

We know the damage that eating too fast can do to our waistline, and if you combine this with the damaging effects of the sugar that is in the majority of calorie-loaded drinks, you get a double-whammy of terribleness for your health and results.

Each time you drink calories, think to yourself: *"My stomach is getting bigger."*

Artificial sweeteners have a similar effect to sugar-loaded liquids because your brain can't discern the difference between the sweet from sugar and artificial sweet. As a result of your brain's confusion, the hormonal response ends up being the same or worse.

Start weaning yourself off of liquid calories and watch the fat melt from your frame. Stick with water, unsweet tea and black coffee.

8. Don't Snack—Snacking Is The Bane Of Weight Loss

One of the reasons Intermittent Fasting is so effective at controlling body composition is because it regulates hormone levels by balancing your body between the "fasted" and "fed" states. In the simplest terms, your body is designed to burn fat when in the *fasted* state and store calories when in the *fed* state. Each time you eat a calorie, you enter the fed state and your body's ability to burn fat is "shut off" by the corresponding release of insulin and glucose floating around your bloodstream.

The next time you grab a bag of almonds thinking it's a healthy snack, think again—you are likely doing more harm than good.

Save calories for mealtime. This will help you avoid the hormone "spikes" that are keeping you fat and sick (and for some, crazy).

9. Take A High-Quality Fish Or Cod Liver Oil With Every Meal

If your meal includes a high-quality omega-3 food source like salmon, sardines, mackerel, grass-fed beef, lamb or bison, then skip the caps for that meal, as you'll already be getting plenty from your food. Your other meals should usually include a dose of omega-3 to help balance out the omega-3 to 6 ratio that is overwhelmingly prevalent in our industrialized food supply.

The food we eat nowadays is a mere fraction of the quality it used to be when we consumed food from the wild. Industrialization produces food that is lacking one way or another. The most prevalent of the nutritional "imbalances" that are the result of mass-produced and processed food, is the fatty acid profiles found in industrialized animal products.

The prevalence of omega-3 and omega-6 fatty acids in nature occurs on a one-to-one scale, on average. Any food high in omega-3s is ideal because the majority of food we eat in this country—and most industrialized food supplies—contain an overwhelming abundance of omega-6. Eating too much omega-6, and not enough omega-3, throws the balance in your body from a one-to-one ratio, as nature intended, completely out of whack. For example, industrialized chicken fat (think crispy, yummy skin) can sport an omega-6 to omega-3 ratio of 8-1. Talk about skewing the numbers.

Try to eat plenty of foods high in omega-3 such as fatty fish and grass-fed red meats like bison, beef and lamb. Also, pastured eggs and butter (Kerrygold is the best) should be staples in your diet.

The next time you eat food high in omega-6, add some extra omega-3 to your meal in pill or food form (food preferred) to help tilt the scale back towards nature's ratio.

10. Take Vitamin D Or Get Sunlight Every Day

Vitamin D is fast becoming the "miracle" supplement because of continuing research that keeps pointing to how essential it is to human health. Humans naturally produce vitamin D from sunlight, typically after 20-30 minutes of exposure. But what happens when you aren't getting sun? Well, you can get a little bit from your food—namely leafy green veggies—but it's just not enough. The amount your body produces in response to getting sunlight is mountains higher than what you can get from food. Basically...

Everyday sunlight is essential to being a healthy human.

For days you can't get outside for at least 20 minutes, pop 5k IU of vitamin D to help keep your levels up. Just make sure you don't substitute the supplement for getting outside on a regular basis. For optimal health, you must regularly bask under the rays of the single star in our solar system (that's the sun, btw).

11. Reduce Stress

Did you know that each time you freak out about something (induce stress) it's like taking a bite out of a candy bar—hormonally speaking?

I once had a client that did everything right. She ate Paleo, trained hard and consistent at least 5 days a week and slept 7-8 hours a night. While she got stronger and fitter, she couldn't lose body fat and lean out, which was her primary goal. The reason? She was a mega-worrier that was always stressed about work and school (and her weight). The moral of this short story is: stress is the Antichrist to your fat and weight loss efforts.

When you are stressed, or become stressed, your body responds by raising cortisol levels. Cortisol is a stress hormone used primarily in the "fight or flight" response we default to in times of physical danger—also known as the "stress response." Short bouts of stress are useful for keeping us "on our toes" and safe from danger, but chronic stress, as is so prevalent in our modern society, is a slow killer.

Chronic stress results in chronically elevated cortisol levels, which in turn breaks down muscle mass, halts fat-loss, promotes fat-gain and screws up your overall health to epic proportions.

It's time to take a chill pill and relax. Be patient. Give yourself a break. You don't have to be perfect. Don't be afraid of messing up and making mistakes; that's how you learn. In fact, you should embrace it as par for the course. If you aren't making mistakes, you probably aren't doing very much. Change your perception of reality and you have the power to mitigate the mountain of stress that is ruining your health and weight loss efforts.

Find ways to reduce the stress in your life. Some ways to reduce stress include mindfulness, meditation, taking a walk, counting your breath, spending time with friends and family, spending time in nature, exercise, and so on.

Stress is a killer of your own doing. Stress is like being prescribed the pill of death by doctor Kevorkian, then saying "Ok thanks" before proceeding to take your daily dose every day with the knowledge that you are killing yourself. It's time to stop that.

You decide how you respond to the world. You can stress out about the million things you can't control, or you can sit back, kick your feet up, and take comfort in the fact that you are lucky to be alive and that everything else is just pure, thick, gluten-free, gravvvvvy.

12. Eat High-Quality Animal Products

Keywords for quality food include: grass-fed, free-range, pastured, organic, all-natural, hormone-free, humanely raised, family farms, local.

Protein from healthy animals should comprise about 20-40% of your total calorie intake (more for those of you trying to pack on muscle). The easiest way to start tracking your protein intake is to make sure you are eating at least a handful-sized amount each meal. Protein should cover about 1/3 of your plate—the rest comprised of fat, and, to a lesser extent, carbs.

Examples include: a piece of fish, a steak, 1-2 pieces of chicken, a mound of grass-fed beef, and a mound of scrambled eggs.

13. Eat High-Quality Fat

Most people think fat is "bad." They're wrong. There are a few fats that are "bad" like trans fat, soybean oil, vegetable oil, and seed oils. Then there are fats that are ok in moderation such as nut oils and unheated olive oil. Finally, there are fats you should be eating every day as a staple in your diet. These include: fatty fish, grass-fed beef, lamb and bison, coconut, pastured butter (Kerrygold is the best), avocados, and ghee (from grass-fed milk).

Your body requires a healthy dose of what's known as "essential fatty acids," notably the omega-3 and omega-6 fatty acids we covered in number 9. "Essential" means we must get them from outside sources or we will die because our body doesn't produce them. The same is true of the essential amino acids found in protein. (There are no "essential" carbohydrates in nature. Tells you something about the importance of fat and protein over carbohydrates, doesn't it?)

Fat provides more fuel per gram than protein and carbs—perhaps part of the reason it's our body's preferred fuel source.

The breakdown goes like this:

Fat = 9 calories per 1 gram
Protein = 4 calories per 1 gram
Carb = 4 calories per 1 gram
Alcohol = 7 calories per 1 gram (yup)

Fat burns more evenly than carbs and protein—both of which are fickle fuel sources. Another thing about fat, which is the paradox that often confuses people, is it doesn't trigger fat gain the way eating carbohydrates, and, to a lesser extent, protein does. This has to do with our hormones. The most prevalent hormone that triggers fat gain is insulin. Insulin is linked to the raising of blood sugar levels as a result of eating carbohydrates. Because carbohydrates result in the greatest release of insulin upon ingesting, it is most often correlated with fat gain.

Fat, on the other hand, is hormonally neutral, meaning it doesn't spike hormones when you eat it. Fat actually provides a "buffer" effect that helps regulate the levels of your hormones when you eat protein and/or carbs (and why you should eat some every meal).

Fat review:

- Fat has more energy per gram and fuels your body more effectively than carbs or protein
- Fat helps buffer hormone levels when eating carbs and protein (always eat some with your meals)
- Fat doesn't cause wild fluctuations in your hormones the way carbs do
- Fat includes omega-3 and omega-6 fatty acids which are essential to life
- Fat is damn tasty
- Fat triggers the "full" feeling (carbs tend to trigger "eat more")

14. Perform Resistance Training An Average Of Three Times A Week

You probably already know why this is beneficial, so *just do it*.

Men and women alike should be utilizing strength training as an integral part of their fitness program. My book "The Gym Life Book Of Fitness" will teach you everything you need to know about utilizing a strength program and building world-class general fitness.

Let's review some of the benefits of resistance training:

It "tightens" everything up: less jiggle, more firmness, more tone.
It makes your body look proportional.
No more "chicken legs" or "turkey arms."
In the immortal words of Mark Rippetoe, "It makes you harder to kill and more useful in general."
Muscle protects you from death, decay and disease.

It strengthens ligaments and joints.
It prevents atrophy from aging.

Muscle gives your body a better chance at fighting off all the nasty things trying to infect and kill you (disease, parasites, viruses, trauma). It will even help you survive an accident better than someone with less muscle mass. It really is our *natural body armor*.

For guys, I don't have to say much: it's almost universal that men want to build more muscle and strength. However, for women, this isn't true. And that's a bloody shame. This is often due to the misconception that lifting weights will make a woman "big" or "bulky." This is a valid concern, sure. *It's just not a practical one.* The majority of women, I'd say about 99.9999% of you, don't have the genetic make-up to ever have to even worry about getting big or bulky. And as a hypothetical, let's say you start training and you started seeing you were getting *bigger*. What would you do?

> *You would slow down, change your program or stop*
> *altogether... right?*

So really, what are you worried about? Muscle doesn't grow overnight. It takes months and years to develop muscle mass... especially the kind that anyone would ever consider "big." Furthermore, it's your diet that determines how big you'll get. If you don't want to get big, eat well and you won't.

That said, you should at least try it out for yourself. Brushing it off by saying you are afraid of getting big because you've seen women online that are big (many of whom take drugs, train hours a day, and have been doing both for years), **is just an excuse**. And this excuse will result in an early and unnecessary death.

If you want the best chance at beating cancer, heart disease, and the countless accidental and internal ways you can die fast or slow, than you must make strength training a priority. *Or not.* Either way, you will reap what you sow. End Sermon.

A simple template for resistance training sessions:

1. **Main lift:** Shoulder Press at a 5x5 rep scheme
2. **1st accessory set:** 3-5 sets of Handstand pushups (or max effort holds)
3. **2nd accessory:** Ring or bar dips for 3-5 reps, adding weight each set
4. **3rd accessory:** A dumbbell exercise like DB push-presses or bodyweight like one-arm push-ups
5. **Second Main lift:** Bench press or squats or deadlift (or skip if you are lifting more days and targeting one big lift per session)
6. **1st accessory** for 2nd big lift
7. **2nd accessory** for 2nd big lift
8. **3rd accessory** for 2nd big lift
9. **Skill work** for 10-15 minutes
10. **Conditioning** for 5-20 minutes
11. **Cool-down**
12. **Go home and feel good**
13. **Wake up and look and feel *sexier***

15. Eliminate Sugar

Sugar is the absolute worst thing you can eat (besides maybe molten lava... and even then... I'm not so sure).

As we discussed above, fat does not make you fat. Sugar, refined grains, processed food, white starches, seed oils and synthetics are what make you fat. These "foods" wreak havoc on the internals of your body. They confuse your brain, cause your hormones to do the funky chicken dance and promote the silent killer known as inflammation.

Barry Spears, the founder of the Zone diet, coined the term "silent inflammation" to describe the internal damage that results from internal stressors in the body, the most notable being food and its effect on your hormones.

The Zone diet is based on controlling hormones by balancing carbohydrates, proteins and fats via a system known as the "block system." By eating a certain number of "blocks" each day, you are regulating the amount of carbs, protein and fat you consume. *It works.* It was actually the first "diet" I ever got results with.

The problem I now have with the Zone diet is the lack of focus on food quality. Zone is largely focused on controlling the amounts of food you eat while focusing less on the quality of the food. Some people coin this "Cheeseburger Zone" in which people eat junk food but eat it within the confines of the "block" system and think it's going to help them. Of course, I'm sure Dr. Spears probably encourages eating whole, real foods but I can't comment on that. I'm just reporting on what I've seen and what led me astray when I was following the diet myself.

My point in sharing this with you is to highlight the importance of hormones and how controlling your carbohydrate intake is integral to optimal health and weight loss. Your meals should include a balanced amount of fat, protein and carbs. And as the Zone diet suggests through its block system—which I concur with—you should take a low-carb approach.

Fundamentally, the Western diet is high-carb, low-fat and moderate protein. One reason America is fat and sick is we are addicted to carbs, mostly sugar and grains. If you take the complications that sugars and grains cause and combine it with the problems that eating too many carbohydrates produce before finally tacking on the lack of nutrition inherent in a high-carb diet as the result of not eating enough quality protein and fat, you end up with a recipe for disaster. Disaster in this case ends up as heart disease, diabetes, obesity, cancer, and every other totally preventable modern disease.

This is a calling to completely change your view of what nutrition is. When you eliminate sugar and grains, you end up removing most processed foods as a result. Of course, this can be brutally hard. They say sugar is more addictive than cocaine, and it's in EVERYTHING. I've never done cocaine, but I can tell you right now that I still battle with sugar cravings on a daily basis, and I eat better than most people I know.

Start doing this: read labels and avoid all foods that contain the ingredient "sugar" (or grains). Other examples of sugar that are touted on labels as something else are: cane sugar, high fructose corn syrup, rice syrup, corn syrup, fructose, evaporated cane juice, cane syrup, and agave nectar (no, this is not a healthy sweetener).

16. Perform High-Intensity Interval Training ~3x a week

Also known as "HIIT" training, the premise of high-intensity interval (or intermittent) training is based on completing work against the clock—or *how fast you complete an allotted amount of work*. The faster you perform a task, the more power you generate and the greater the level of intensity your body produces. For fat loss, muscle building, and overall fitness improvement, HIIT training is brutally effective.

If you haven't already noticed the meteoritic rise rising of interval-based circuit training in popular fitness literature, then I'm here to tell you that it's here to stay. And this is good. The old ways of training—bodybuilding and steady-state cardio—which do very little for the majority of people, are finally losing the popular vote.

The three principles of HIIT training revolve around time, distance and movement. The fundamental goal of HIIT training is to move a load the longest possible distance in the shortest amount of time. This is represented by the "Power" formula: Force x Distance / Time = power output. Power is measured in joule per second; more commonly referred to as "watts," after James Watt, the inventor of the steam engine. The basic premise of the power formula, as it applies to mechanical human fitness, is the more power you generate the greater you improve your fitness. Or simply put: higher intensity = improved fitness.

To visualize the power formula, consider the difference between running a mile and sprinting 100m for time. Running a mile at a 6 or 7 minute pace will result in a more intense effort than running a 10-minute mile but significantly less intensity than an all-out 100-meter sprint.

Think of the last time you trained something long(er) distance. Now think about the last time you did something as fast as you could. The former was invariably at an easier, slower pace while the latter was at a frantic, sweat dripping, giving-everything-you-got, kind of pace. Do you see the power equation at play? When you sprint, you move your body as fast as you can until the race is complete. When you run a marathon, you pace yourself so you are able to finish because an all-out sprint would be physically impossible to sustain and result in you burning out before the finish line.

To develop total fitness, you should train many speeds and distances. You should sprint, train endurance, and target everything between those two ends of the spectrum. But when it comes to fat loss, and developing the greatest adaptation in the least amount of time possible, **training at your highest intensities should comprise the bulk of your conditioning efforts**.

The main reason you want to root your training in high-intensity effort is because of the effect this modality has on the other, *slower*, modalities. For example, it has been proven that short intervals of high-intensity exercise can increase VO2 max, which in turn makes you better at medium and long distance training (See: The Tabata Study).

Fundamentally, training high-intensity is the most effect way to improving overall fitness. A great way to illustrate the difference in athletes that use predominately high-intensity training vs. long-distance and/or steady-state training is the popular picture showcasing an Olympic sprinter vs. an Olympic endurance runner. Do this: Google "sprinter vs. marathon runner picture" and check out the top three results. I'd provide you the link, but I want you to take the effort yourself so you are more likely to remember what you see (and ingrain the difference in your mind).

To produce speed, your body must generate large amounts of power. This requires muscle mass.

Moving a weight for long distances requires a constant supply of energy. While your body can use up fat stores to fuel this activity, it will also utilize muscle mass. In fact, it might be inclined to use muscle *before* fat. Let's see why. We'll use the long-distance runner as an example. When running long distances, muscle mass is a hindrance because it is heavy and must be "dragged" along. As a result, the body will want to remove this "dead weight" as a means of better adapting to the physical task at hand. This is a survival mechanism known as homeostasis, in which the body is adapting to external conditions as a means to regulate and survive.

Your body is an adaptive, intelligent machine that operates with a fundamental directive: *survive*. The very reason HIIT exercise produces muscle mass and increased fitness is the same reason muscle wastes away from long-distance exercise when no rest is available: because your body is undergoing stress and is seeking to adjust to the external environment in whatever means that will produce the best chance of survival.

When you train intermittently (alternating between rest and work periods), your body learns that more muscle mass is beneficial to completing the task at hand because it can produce more power and gets short bouts of rest that allow the muscles to partially recuperate before going again. As a result, your body tries to preserve and grow muscle mass compared to endurance training where your body tries to shed muscle. Additionally, HIIT training does not last a long time—somewhere between 5 and 25 minutes—which allows for rest long before your body will start to look to muscle mass for fuel.

Of course, there are other factors that weigh in each of these processes, but it is beyond the scope of this book to delve into them. I suggest you do research on your own if you want to fully understand them. Either way, you should be utilizing high-intensity training in your program on a regular basis. It's right next to resistance training in importance for developing your global fitness.

I implore you to change your mind about what you think steady-state and long-distance modalities are doing for your health and fitness. They are not "calorie-burning" activities that are the key to burning fat, like many think. In fact, study after study, and the mountains of anecdotal evidence we find from the likes of athletes around the world, all point to the fact that HIIT style of training produces a better increase to fitness and faster fat-loss when compared to other modalities. Some food for thought.

Here is a sample training week that can give you an idea of how to incorporate HIIT training into a balanced program.

A Hypothetical Training Week:

Monday: Squats followed by a sled-conditioning workout. 15 minutes of skill work at a moderate pace. A short 5-minute set of max-effort kettlebell swings.
Tuesday: Play a pick-up basketball game. A 20-minute walk after dinner. A few sets of push-ups and stretching at home.

Wednesday: Bench press and upper body accessory work. Complete 10x 50m sprints at 90-100% effort. Yoga for 15 minutes as a cool-down.
Thursday: Walk on the beach. Relax and smell the roses. This is known as a "rest day."
Friday: Warm-up and 30 minute HIIT workout known as a "chipper" of 10 exercises.
Saturday: Lifting session of deadlift, Olympic weightlifting work, and GHD sit-ups. Beach volleyball, jog a couple miles on beach, enjoy a hard-earned cheat meal.
Sunday: Five-mile bike ride at a leisurely pace. Spend two hours prepping food for week. Do 100 push-ups, sit-ups, and squats at home at a slow-medium pace.

Above is an example of what my average training week looks like. Athletes training for a sport will utilize more volume and gym-based sessions than I do. More advanced trainees might choose to train in the gym 5-7 days a week depending on their goals. Of course this is all based on goals and level of fitness.

Personally, I seek a long-term, balanced approach to my fitness. I train so I can be fit and prepared, to look and feel good, and so I can live a long life with plenty of energy. Based on these goals, a less volume, more balanced approach suits me well. The last 13 years I've been training, I've figured out that my body does better with less in-the-gym-volume and more outdoor, gymnastic, and Primal-style training. By mixing my efforts among these various modalities, my body does better. I've learned what works for me and I stick to that. What works for you will be different. The key is to figure it out for yourself.

For those of you that just want to be healthy and look good in the mirror, start here:

Train 2-3 times a week in the gym with high intensity in weightlifting and HIIT conditioning. Between your gym sessions, slip in low-to-moderate intensity activities—get outdoors, move often, walk a lot, stretch and work mobility.

Eat a real food Paleo-based diet. Enjoy time with friends and family. Laugh a lot and be in the moment.

Follow the template above and listen to your body and you can't go wrong. If you choose to sacrifice your health for performance, just make sure you know what you are doing. Avoid falling into the thinking that being "ripped" or "lean" automatically means you are healthy. It's what the inside looks like that determines your health.

17. Practice Mindfulness And Meditation

Our hormones get all out of whack when our racing mind is constantly bombarded with worry, stress, anger, resentment, jealousy, and all the other crap that consumes our thoughts. This is known as "chronic stress," and it's a silent killer (recommended reading: Why Zebras Don't Get Ulcers).

Meditation is the practice of emptying the mind. The simplest form of meditation is to "count your breath." Count "one" each time you breathe in and out. Then count "two" for each breath, then three, etc. By focusing on your breath, you can control, and quiet, your racing mind. This hyper-active, always bouncing from thought to thought, racing mind is what most of us live with, and have no control over, every second of the day. Meditation is a form of taming this beast.

The more you meditate, the more you can silence, or slow down, your thoughts at will. Obviously, focusing on anything is a form of meditation (called mindfulness) and you should aim to do it as much as possible. This is often called *being in the moment.* You are seeing, hearing and experiencing only what is in front of you in the moment. Instead of thinking about something in the past or future, you are in the Now.

You can meditate anywhere.

I like to count my breath while driving. I also take 3-5 minute meditation breaks after every 55 minutes of work in which I'll count my breath and empty my mind. Like anything else, the key is practice. Meditation is mental training just as squats are physical training.

When you meditate, your mind will constantly fight you. It will bring up random thoughts in an attempt to distract you and to take back control. When you find yourself veering from your breath, refocus and get back to the count. This will happen throughout the process. Don't get discouraged, as many do, just keep returning to your breath/count.

It's not about perfection, it's training.

Just as you lift a weight to train the muscles in your body, you meditate to train your mind to be more focused and controlled. Some say that accomplishing a few minutes of pure "emptiness" can take months of training. Keep that in mind with your practice. You aren't seeking perfection.

Mindfulness is the act of doing what you are doing fully without outside thoughts from your distracted mind. Mindfulness is a form of meditation and meditation is a form of mindfulness. The main difference, from my understanding, is meditation is the act of being still and focused for the sake of completely clearing the mind whereas mindfulness is the act of doing something with intense, non-distracted focus.

When you do anything, make it your goal to do only that thing. When you talk on the phone, pay attention to your conversation. Your conversations will get better. When you eat, turn off the music, TV and your phone, and focus on the food. Your food will taste better. When you hang out with friends and family, give them your full attention. Be interested in them. Stay off your phone or in mental outer space. They'll love you more.

Nearly every possible benefit you can attribute to your health, effectiveness, work and relationships can be improved with mediation and mindfulness. I highly, highly, highly recommend you do some more research and start a basic practice. This is life-changing stuff.

Remember, a few minutes a day done at random times can be life changing. You don't have to buy special pillows or sit with folded legs in monk robes to practice and reap the benefits. You could put this book down right now and count 10 breaths. This will steady your breath and quiet your mind. You'd be one step closer to being more in control, less stressed and hurried, and a bit happier. This is how accessible—and powerful—these concepts are.

Recommend: The Power of Now Book, Headspace App

18. Walk As Much As Possible

There is a Chinese proverb that goes like this: "After a meal, walk a hundred steps to live to be ninety-nine."

Walking after a meal is not the only time you should walk— although it's the first place you can start to develop the habit. Our hunter-gatherer ancestors used to walk an average of 13 miles a day. Basically, as humans, we are made to move... and a lot. Daily actives for a hunter-gatherer included gathering, forging, climbing and crawling in search of food. Hunting included moving for long distances coupled with brief periods of sprinting when going in for the kill (looks at bit like interval training, huh?).

The average American walks 2-3 miles a day. This is a fraction of what our ancestors did. Western society doesn't move enough. The easiest way to start moving more is walking.

Start looking for the longest route, not the shortest. When you find yourself driving around the parking lot to find a "close" spot, stop yourself. This is a great time to park at the end of the parking lot and get some walking in (and it'll protect your freaking car doors!). Start parking as far away as possible. Take the stairs. While the *drones* take the escalator, you take the stairs.

Your new mindset should be finding the longest and hardest path.

19. Get Outdoors And Utilize Low-Intensity Movement

We have lived, and moved, in nature for hundreds of thousands of years. It was only the last 10,000 years or so that brought the prevalence of living in permanent structures (around the same time agriculture was introduced). We are not made to live in climate-controlled boxes that limit our movement. We are made to breathe fresh air, hear the sounds of nature (studies show this improves health), touch the earth and nature (known as earthing), and move over uneven, soft and varied terrain on a regular basis.

Try to get outdoors and move as often as possible. This is the perfect way to take an active rest day and get some calorie burning in without infringing on your recovery.

Examples of moving outdoors:
Take a walk after meals
Walk for 5, 10, or 30 minutes
Park at the end of the parking lot
Take the stairs
Walk your dog
Take the longest and least convenient route on purpose
Circle a place a few times before going in
And on and on and on and on

Forms of low-intensity training:
Any endurance based training
Walking
Mobility work
Skill work
Sled work
Hiking
Biking
Swimming
Jogging
Climbing

There is a ton of research that points to the positive health benefits of spending time in nature. Get outdoors and soak it up.

20. Play Sports

Humans love to play games and compete; it's in our DNA. Some of us are more competitive than others, but nonetheless, competition is a trait built into our species from thousands of years of survival. Sports challenge your body to move in non-linear planes that utilize movement patterns not often targeted in a gym setting.

Sports are a great addition to your general fitness program, and best of all, they are fun. The hardest part of fitness is sticking with it; so naturally, anything that makes fitness fun gets two HUGE thumbs up in my book. Play sports because they are fun and they improve your fitness.

Ways to play:
Go to the park
Play pickup games at the field or court
Join a sports league
Bring a football, soccer ball, Frisbee or paddleboard to the beach

Try racquetball (my favorite sport)

Examples of play include:
Running
Jumping
Balancing
Climbing
Swimming
Hand balancing

Places to play:
Parks
Fields
Forest
Jungle
Beach
Mountain
Hill
Trees
Playgrounds
Trails

Sports and games:
Flag football
Dodgeball
Baseball
Kickball
Tennis
Obstacle courses/races
Kayaking
Surfing
Paddle-boarding
Etc.

Download the 20 Ways to Live A Healthy Lifestyle Poster (and the Gym Life Files bundle pack) here: www.GymLifeClub.com

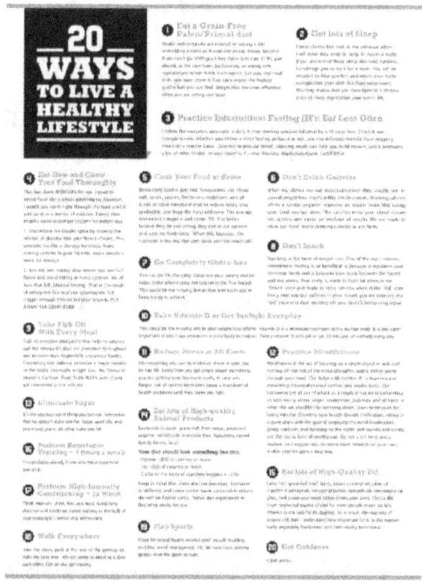

We just covered the main 20 ways to promote health and fitness in your life. Try to attack these before spending too much energy on the other 30. The rest of the techniques for losing weight are still useful, and will help you to varying degrees, but if you haven't already adopted the first 20, you won't be getting the best ROI for your time spent.

Focus on 1-20 for the initial 80% or so of your results. Then when you get stuck at a plateau, start experimenting with the other tips to help you bust through.

If you have any questions or comments about any of this, shoot me an email: ismynamecolin@gmail.com. I'm here to help.

More Tips for Weight Loss

21. Drink Green Tea

Green tea is full of antioxidants and a bit of caffeine—both good for fat burning. I use a variety of different tea like white, black, green, fruity and chocolate. I drink them unsweet, and sometimes with a lemon or lime wedge. I also prefer them iced.

I keep the following tea in my cabinet:

Green
Yerba Mate
Black
White fruity teas: pear, berry, etc.
Cocoa (yum)

22. Train High-Intensity

Everyone can and should do some form of high-intensity training. There are many ways to do it—you can do more WODs, less WODs, strength-bias, endurance-bias, gymnastics-bias, competition focused, etc. It's a great program for developing GPP (general physical preparedness) and it makes fitness fun.

There's a lot of "hate" surrounding HIIT, but it's all hogwash. Most of these misinformed opinions come from fitness professionals that feel threatened because their training methods are becoming obsolete, and from athletes stuck in their own dogma that are too afraid to "open up" to other forms of training. It's all nonsense.

Try it for yourself and you'll see.

To start, I recommend trying a free class at each box in your area. Each gym is going to have its own feel, so you should find one that fits you. No matter what you start training, you <u>must</u> take it slow and learn the movements. This will prevent you from doing something stupid like injuring yourself then blaming the method.

23.Take ZMA or Other Magnesium Supplement Before Bed

ZMA is hands down my favorite supplement. It contains zinc, magnesium and vitamin B-6. It helps you sleep deeper and recover faster. Magnesium is a vital mineral that aids in weight loss and a host of other bodily functions—one of which is appetite regulation. Women are especially susceptible to being defunct in both magnesium and zinc.

If you have yet to start a supplement routine, make ZMA your first. You won't be disappointed. Plus, as far as supplements go, it's pretty cheap.

My three favorite products: Natural Stacks MagTech, Natural Calm, ZMA by Now Foods

24. Watch Your Carb Intake

This includes sugar, rice, potatoes, fruit, alcohol, and grains (hopefully you aren't eating grains). As we've covered, carbs should represent the lowest percentage of your daily calorie intake—somewhere between 20-30%.

Ideally, you want your carb intake to be made of starchy and fibrous vegetables and sweet potatoes/yams. Avoid sugar at all costs.

25. Fast Before You Train— And Sometimes After

The longer you go without food in your body, the more your body will utilize stored fat for energy (also known as 'burning fat'). When you train, your body's fuel needs raise exponentially. After your body burns up the available glucose in your body, it will turn to fat stores for energy. If you introduce glucose into your body after eating calories, you limit your body's ability to utilize fat stores. Obviously, this isn't ideal for burning fat or losing weight.

Fasting helps keep your glucose low so your body can quickly burn what is left before moving into the fat burning state.

I always train on an empty stomach, or as it's more commonly known, "in the fasted state." For many of you, this might take some getting used to, especially if you are used to eating before your workouts, but if you give it some time, I promise it'll be worth it.

You can also fast post-workout from time to time to mix things up. This technique is especially powerful if you are trying to lose weight (although not always ideal if you are lean and trying to build muscle).

Start fasting before you train. Your performance will improve drastically.

26. Get Social

Human beings are social animals that have thrived for thousands of years by staying together. Our ancestors lived as hunter gathers in close-knit tribes of 40-80 people. Members of a tribe shared all resources with one another. During this time, humans had no concept of personal property. The tribe was like a big family, and there was no reason to own anything on a personal level (being greedy could even get you kicked out of the tribe and forced to fend for yourself in the harsh wild). Compare this to the greedy, self-centered, and guarded nature of humans nowadays.

We are made to share our lives with other people. It's built into our DNA. No matter how introverted you prefer to be, your happiness levels will always suffer as a result. Invest time into your personal relationships, and you will be amazed at the positive effect it will have on your health and results (and happiness).

27. Utilize "Active Rest" Days

There are times when your body isn't recovered enough from your previous training session. When this happens, putting in more work (stress) would be counter-productive to your results. This is the perfect time for an "active rest" day. An active rest day utilizes low-intensity exercise and recovery protocols like skill and mobility work.

When training active rest, throttle the volume, speed and intensity depending on how sore you are from your previous session. Remember, you don't want to cut into your recovery and risk overtraining.

This is a great time to work weaknesses, flexibility, or for training an underdeveloped modality like swimming, running or rowing.

Some of my favorite ways to train active rest include:

- Light rowing
- Olympic weightlifting technique work
- Handstands and gymnastics skill work with lots of rest
- Mobility and foam rolling
- Getting outdoors and moving
- Practicing skills and drills for a sport

Active rest days are a great way to get a bit of exercise and work on some skills without cutting into your recovery.

28. Do Nothing (Strategically)

There are days you should lie around like a fat, lazy Jabba The Hutt (granted you aren't one). This will relieve mental and physical stress, both of which will provide a massive benefit to your results. This recommendation will come easy to some of you and not so easy to others. Make sure you use this technique strategically. You don't want to fall into the habit of doing nothing *too often* (obviously).

For those that are constantly "go, go, go," this will do wonders for you. If you already have an ample dose of "lazy" built into your routine, try doing a bit of *something* instead of *nothing*, like taking a walk.

Examples of doing nothing include:
Mindless TV, movies, people watching, tanning at the beach, napping, reading, and anything else that isn't too physically demanding.

29. Add 10 "Chews" Each Mouthful

I know, chewing again. Well, it's that important. Chewing improves digestion in multiple ways (as we've covered). The better you digest food, the less you'll feel that annoying "lethargic" feeling after eating, and the more your body will utilize the nutrition in food to repair and grow.

30. Make Things Difficult... On Purpose

Always take the longest route. Carry as many groceries as possible. Run the stairs instead of walking them. Lunge to your car. Climb something. Walk around the building twice before going in.

Move All The Time.

Seek to find ways to always move and challenge yourself. Start doing a bit here and there, and at the end of the year you'll have burned thousands of calories and see a real improvement in the mirror. Fitness is a long game. Never forget that.

31. Buy Some Weightlifting Shoes (or Chuck Taylor's)

When you move heavy weight, it's ideal to have a flat and solid surface to train on. By lifting on a solid, stable base, your body is more efficient at lifting weight—and safer. The more weight you move, the more calories you burn, and the more muscle you build.

Get a pair of lifting shoes. It'll make a big difference.

32. Sprint Once A Week

Fast, intense, full-body exercise like sprinting has profound thermogenic and EPOC effects on the body. It basically turns your body into a calorie-burning furnace during, and after, you train. This is exactly why building muscle is more effective at burning calories than other forms of *cardio*.

Sprinting builds strong legs that are the epitome of functional. Plus, you'll get faster, which could save your life someday.

33. Eat Hot And Hearty Soups And Stews

Soups and stews are filling. Eat them HOT and slow. They are a great way to add variety to your diet.

34. Eat Healthy Fat 15 Minutes Before Meals

Fat triggers a release of hormones that signal to your brain that you are "full." Kick start these hormones by nibbling on some nuts, seeds, organic dark chocolate (70% or higher), or other clean fat source before meals. This will prevent over-eating and aid in calorie-restriction.

35. Perform Heavy, Complex, Functional Movements

When you train your body as a whole, you burn more calories by utilizing more muscles. For those of you stuck in "isolation land," I implore you to start picking up, carrying, and moving heavy objects on a regular basis. Always think: Go big and compound or go home.

36. Avoid Liquid Food

Yes, this includes protein shakes. Drinking calories causes a larger-than-normal insulin spike compared to eating your food whole because of the speed that the calories enter your body. Since insulin is a storage hormone, you want to limit and regulate it as much as possible. An abundance of insulin causes fat gain and a host of other problems in your body.

If you are trying to lose weight, you should avoid drinking calories in any form.

Liquid food also circumvents the chewing process, which is integral to digestion and the release of digestive enzymes. In fact, anytime you have a smoothie or juice, try to "chew" as you drink. This will help release some of these digestive enzymes.

If you do opt for a shake or juice, at the very least you should drink it slow. This will control how fast the calories enter your blood stream.

37. Skip The Condiments (Or Make Homemade Versions)

When I cut ketchup (and milk) out of my diet, I shed the last 5-10 pounds of belly fat I had been struggling with for months. Ketchup and most other condiments are bad news for your waistline. A serving of ketchup, which is 2 tbsp, contains 4 grams of sugar. Plus, there is little to NO nutritional benefit to ketchup (and the marketing claims of lycopene or whatever are pure nonsense).

Store-bought condiments are laden with sugar, preservatives, seed and vegetables oils, and all kinds of other crap. Avoid them and make your own at home.

Small tweaks to your diet like this might not seem like a big deal, but keep in mind that many small tweaks add up to a larger whole. It's often the culmination of these many small habits that is the difference between those with abs and those without.

Make your own condiments. My favorites include: Paleo sriracha, Paleo ketchup, and Paleo BBQ sauce.

38. Take A Digestive Enzyme, Probiotic, And Eat Fermented Foods Regularly

Examples of fermented foods include Kim chi, sauerkraut, kefir, and kombucha. I'd stay away from the yogurt and other products marketed as "probiotics." There might be some that are reasonable quality, but from what I have seen, these are just sugar-laden containers of yogurt made from crappy milk.

Your gut is often said to be the "window" to your health. It's where nutrition goes before being used by your body. We all know how important vitamins and minerals are, so it makes sense that the access we have to them—through digestion—the healthier we are. A lack of access to specific vitamins, minerals, fats and amino acids can cause a host of problems in your health and put a major damper on your weight-loss efforts.

39. Drink Black Coffee (In Moderation)

Coffee offers many benefits to the body, one of which is fat burning, but there are caveats. I recommend sticking with 1 to 2 cups of coffee a day, and to cycle your habits every few weeks with a few days off. Personally, I like to skip a day once or twice a week so I don't develop a habit—and to sensitize myself to the caffeine.

Coffee beans are one of the most heavily sprayed crops in the world. Always opt for Organic and Fair Trade beans. My favorite brand is Bulletproof Coffee. I use it every morning to make the Butter Coffee recipe. (It's amazing.)

40. Eat Protein And Fat Before Your Carbs

Protein is very satiating; it fills you up fast. Fat is also satiating but not as much as protein. I also find fat a bit too easy to consume (it's so tasty), so if you are watching your calories, you have to be careful here. First start with protein each meal.

41. Drink A Full Glass Of Water Before Each Meal

This will fill you up and you'll eat fewer calories.

42. Drink Water Throughout The Day

You don't have to drink as much water as the pundits would have you believe, but for reducing cravings, making you feel full before eating, and for hydrating your body, water is useful and necessary. Listen to your thirst; it's there for a reason.

43. Think Hard And Often - Use Your Brain

Your brain is responsible for up to 20% of your body's resting metabolic rate (the amount of energy your body burns when not doing anything). Since your brain's primary fuel source is glucose, the more *you think*, the more glucose you use up. For weight loss, the more glucose you use up, the less likely any left over can be stored as fat. So really: thinking = weight loss.

It's no wonder people try to avoid thinking. Just like exercise, using your brain requires energy. And just like your body, your brain needs exercise on a regular basis or it will atrophy.

Ways to think include puzzles, crosswords, Sudoku, reading, writing, problem solving, brainstorming, creating art.

44. Use Tabata Intervals

A Tabata interval is a 4-minute interval consisting of 20-second work periods followed by 10-second rest periods. To perform a Tabata interval, pick a movement—air squat for example—and set a timer. For the first 20 seconds, perform as many air squats as possible. Then rest for 10 seconds. Repeat until 4 minutes is complete and you have completed 8 work and rest sets.

The Tabata interval was made famous by Dr. Tabata's research with Olympic speed skaters. He found that athletes utilizing the Tabata interval to train had a 28% increase in VO2 max compared to athletes using only traditional, steady state training. (Link to study: http://www.ncbi.nlm.nih.gov/pubmed/8897392)

I love the Tabata protocol because it gives you a quick workout protocol you can do anytime, anywhere and with no equipment.

How to create a Tabata workout:
Choose an exercise or two
Set timer or stopwatch
Do reps for 20 seconds then rest for 10 Complete 8 rounds

45. Take Naps

Sleep is one of the top 5 prerequisites for living a healthy life. There is a ton of research pointing to the benefits of napping, but for most of you, this doesn't matter because you're already chronically sleep-deprived. For those of you sleep-deprived zombies, napping is even more important of a tool because it'll help you erase some of your "sleep debt."

Get more sleep whenever and however you can. Naps are great for us all.

46. Replace Soda, Juice, And Sweet Drinks with Soda Water, Tea, Or Sparkling water

Use soda water, sparkling water and tea to wean off the addictive drinks full of sugar and calories. Soda water is a great way to replace cravings for carbonation. Add a splash of lime or lemon and you'll quickly develop a taste for it.

Soda water and lime is a great way to "fake it" at the bar or club: you'll still look cool and hip and no one will know you're sipping bubbly water.

47. Choose Gluten-Free Cider Over Gluten-Filled Beer, And Liquor Over Mix Drinks.

Beer is the Antichrist to your abs. So are mix drinks loaded with sugar. A Long Island ice tea has 780 calories and 40 grams of sugar. Holy crap... and to think I used to drink those [smacks forehead].

Try the Paleo Margarita by Robb Wolf: http://paleoblocks.com/paleo-recipe-robb-wolfs-nor-cal-margaritas/

48. Avoid Artificial Sweeteners

These include sucralose (Splenda), aspartame, saccharin, sorbitol, isomalt, glycerol, mailitol and many others that get slipped in under different names (corporations are tricky). If you can't pronounce it, don't eat it.

There are a bunch of studies that point to the many risks associated with consuming artificial sweeteners, but the main reason you'll want to avoid them is because they make you fat. Yup, zero calories and still fattening.

Artificial sweeteners are many times sweeter than table sugar (sucralose is 600 times sweeter). The reason this is bad for you is because your brain can't discern the difference between "fake" sweet and "real" sweet. As a result of your brain's confusion, the hormonal response from consuming artificial sweeteners ends up being the same—or worse—as eating sugar.

Artificial sweeteners also ruin your palate and make you crave more sweet-tasting foods. Further, we don't fully understand the internal damage these chemicals do when passing through the human body... yet.

Avoid them.

49. Don't Overtrain

Avoid overtraining at all costs. It will sap your weight loss efforts, break down your hard-earned muscle mass, ruin your sleep, stress you out, and promote fat gain.

You avoid overtraining by listing to your body and making intelligent decisions with your rest periods and recovery protocols based on the feedback it is giving you. The program you follow should always be thought of as only a set of guidelines, and not a set-in-stone, one-size-fits-all gospel that will work for you the way it may work for others. Your body has its own program. You just have to figure out what that is. Use testing, tweaking and modifying to find your perfect program.

This is a common mistake I see many athletes make. They try to follow the same program—day to day, pound for pound, rep for rep—as some of the world's best athletes. Unless you are competing at the same level, you should never expect to be able to follow advanced programs exactly the way the top athletes do. There is a reason they are the best in the world.

If they aren't already, your sleep and nutrition should be top notch. The weaker you are in these areas, the slower you'll progress. There are no shortcuts here. If you are serious about your results, it should be an easy decision to put in the time eating clean and getting enough sleep.

50. Plan Ahead: Pack Lunch, Slow Cook Meals, Save Leftovers

The best defense is a strong offense.

When you are prepared, you are less likely to slip into old habits. The key to consistency is making it as **easy** as possible.

Making decisions to eat this or that, to train or not train, to sleep or not sleep, and so on, all take energy. This is known as "decision fatigue" and it is the theory—proven by research—that we start each day with a certain amount of decision-making energy and the more we make decisions, no matter how inconsequential, the more of this energy we *deplete*.

This is why you make poor decisions when you are stressed or tired. You simply have less energy (sometimes called 'willpower') left inside to make a better decision.

President Obama has a closet of 7 of the same suit that he wears every day. He does this because, in his own words:

"You'll see I wear only gray or blue suits. I'm trying to pare down decisions. I don't want to make decisions about what I'm eating or wearing. Because I have too many other decisions to make."

Regardless of how you feel about him, he has the right idea.

Utilize this principle in your life by being prepared. Slow cook a meal for the week and portion it into meal-size containers. Then, the next time you don't feel like cooking, reheat one of these containers and congratulate yourself for avoiding another "slip."

Another technique is to set out your gym outfit the night before—doing so will make you more likely to go to the gym because you'll have one less decision to make (research showing this exact technique increased the gym-going rates of people participating in the study as much as 60%). The same goes for putting on your workout shoes.

You can use this technique in all walks of life. Use planning to reduce decision fatigue by making things easy.

Read this article about achieving your goals using two tricks: http://jamesclear.com/implementation-intentions

Great job... Now get to work!

Thanks for reading. I really, really hope you will take action and start implementing some of these techniques into your program. Developing habits can be difficult. Keep this in mind when you are trying to implement these new habits in your life. Be prepared to wax and wane during the process. That's to be expected. Just be patient and consistent. Celebrate consistency, not perfection.

Perfection is a fool's errand

Start small: Pick one or two techniques at a time and do them consistently until they "stick." Then add one or two more and repeat the process. Keep building habit upon habit until you end up with the program that is getting you the results you've always dreamed of!

This crazy thing we call *health and fitness* is all based on our habits. Focus on consistency, not perfection, and you'll get there. Just keep going no matter what.

If you ever need any help or have any questions, please shoot me an email: ismynamecolin@gmail.com

Yours in Fitness,

-Colin Stuckert

Resources

The following section includes quotes and links from the top experts in the world on all things fitness and training. I owe much of my education to them. You should definitely check them out. Also, there is something you should know about fitness:

There are many ways to skin a cat.

Some coaches produce world-class Olympic athletes using one style while others might use a completely different method and still send their athletes to compete for the gold. Keep that in mind the next time someone tells you this is the "only" or "best" way to train. Always test protocols out for yourself. Avoiding buying into any one fitness dogma, and never be closed-minded with your education. *Always be learning.*

Each human body will adapt differently to different forms of training. Some modalities will complement the things you are better at while others might target your weaknesses—and will probably get better results from the latter. Make sense?

I've said it before and I'll say it again: you must figure it out for yourself. You have the best *operational manual* to yourself. No one can tell you what your body is telling you. Listen to it.

Kelly Starrett:
http://www.mobilitywod.com/about/kellystarrett/

Author of Becoming a Supple Leopard and founder of MobilityWod.com

Louie Simmons: http://www.westside-barbell.com

Powerlifting legend and Founder/owner of Westside Barbell and author of numerous books and articles

Mark Rippetoe: http://startingstrength.com

Author of Starting Strength

Mark Sisson: http://marksdailyapple.com

My go-to resource for all things ancestral-based health and nutrition. His site is all you need to learn everything you need to know about optimal health and nutrition.

Dave Asprey: http://www.bulletproofexec.com

The Bulletproof Exec and founder of the wildly successful Bulletproof Radio Podcast. His podcast is a must-listen.

Robb Wolf: http://robbwolf.com

My introduction to Paleo eating when I started out some 5 years ago. Robb is a pioneer of the Paleo movement and his podcast is great.

This short list comprises the majority of resources that have contributed to my education on these topics. You should buy their books, subscribe to their podcasts and newsletters, and support them anyway you can.

Tools

Fasting

Leangains.com
MarksDailyApple.com

Exercise

5/3/1 Program by Jim Wendler

Nutrition

Bulletproofexec.com
Robbwolf.com
MarksDailyApple.com

Tools

A Small Crockpot: This thing is AMAZING; consider getting 2 and loading them up each morning
Big Crockpot: great for bigger meals
Victorinox Chef Knives: Cheapest knives that still provide amazing results
Magic Bullet: I use this thing for my Bulletproof Coffee and protein shakes
Aero Press: Preferred way to brew coffee
French Press: 2nd preferred way to brew coffee. Also great for brewing loose tea
Cast-iron skillets: Last a lifetime; get an 8,10 and 12 inch)
Lacrosse ball: For trigger-point release

Food Ingredients

Bulletproof Coffee
MCT oil

Kerrygold Butter
Himalayan Sea Salt

Supplements

Ciltep By Natural Stacks
Performance Essentials stack by Natural Stacks
ZMA by Now Foods
Vitamin D by Now Foods
Vitamin C by Now Foods

Books

GymLifeCook.com: My book on cooking technique. Learn how to cook meals without the use of recipes by learning basic cooking technique you can use over and over.
GymLifeBooks.com: My library of books to help you become the best version of yourself possible!
Tao of Jeet Kune Do: Bruce Lee is my childhood idol. This book is not just about fighting, it's pack-loaded with philosophy.
The Alchemist: International bestseller.
The Four-Hour Body: Tim Ferris fan. Check out his books.
The Richest Man in Babylon: Great book on money.
The Art of Living: The Classical Manual on Virtue, Happiness, and Effectiveness: This book can change your life. It had a role in changing mine.

About The Author

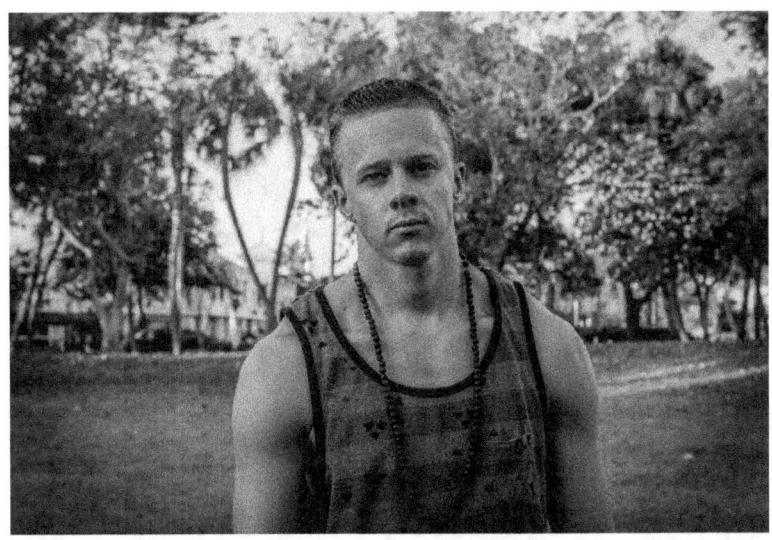

My name is Colin and I'm obsessed with personal development, food and fitness. Like Bruce Lee—my childhood idol—I believe in personal responsibility. What I get in my life is based on me. What you get in your life is based on you. Instead of complaining about the fairness of life and the good luck of others, I'd rather get working and make myself better.

"Time means a lot to me because you see I am also a learner and am often lost in the joy of forever developing."
-Bruce Lee

Of course, this isn't the easiest path. It's much easier to sit on the couch and make excuses. It's hard to do work every day... especially when it feels like you aren't moving anywhere... <u>but this is exactly what it takes</u>.

While others will quit after the grind sets in and their motivation wanes, I'll be plowing through (and I hope you will as well). And this is, in my opinion, what separates the winners from the losers, the wheat from the chaff, the cream to the top, the cat from the mouse, and so on.

What I do for a living

I started my first business in 2009: a juice and smoothie bar located inside a large corporate gym (ironic, I know). I started my second business 8 months later a few miles down the road—The Training Box—a group-fitness and MMA gym. As I'm writing this, it's been 5 and a half years of learning, blood, sweat and tears, more learning, wasting money, making some back, being sued, spending (we call it "reinvestment" but sometimes I'm not so sure of the difference), plenty of stress, more learning, and now here.

I've worked *really* hard to grow my businesses to be as self-sufficient as possible. Recommended book on the subject: The E-Myth Revisited. Since I've been fortunate enough to attract a great group of people to work in my businesses, I now have the freedom of not having to work "in" my businesses, which allows me the time to pursue other passions (like writing). That said, it's still a lot of work. In fact, 95% (maybe more) of what it takes to run a business goes on behind "closed doors."

I went to college for a couple years but didn't do well. I stopping going right before speech class credit was due because I was afraid to speak in front of people (which is ironic considering I've had to use this very skill on a daily basis since I started teaching classes at our Box). *But such is life.* I never did well in school and I was always led to believe that I wasn't "smart" or that I would grow up to be a "loser." That's what they convince you of anyway.

When I discovered that you could work hard in your own business to determine your results, I was hooked. To me, personal development and success in business go hand-in-hand. Actually, I can't imagine being that good at business if you aren't good at making yourself better. It's the "always improving" mindset that succeeds. You have to face challenges head-on and hustle to overcome them—and learn from the lessons so you are better next time.

Of course, there are many people who work hard, neglect their health, and still get results in certain areas of life. The thing is, I believe these poor souls could get much greater results—plus all the benefits of being healthy—if they took a health-first approach. Personally, I'm utterly useless if I'm sick or tired. I just curl up in a little ball and my motivation to do anything disappears. This is why, for me, health always comes first. When I feel my best, I perform my best. When I improve myself, I get better at everything else. *This is my fundamental approach to life.*

I've met many of these not so healthy yet uber-successful people over the years and their situation always perplexes me. What's the point of having money if you can't enjoy it? Is it really worth working 80 hours a week just so you can watch the numbers in your bank account tick upwards? I don't get it.

If it were me, I would be traveling the world and getting into as much adventure as my success could finance. I would spearfish off the coast of Caribbean islands in a chartered boat, scuba dive in Australia near the great barrier reef, surf in Hawaii, climb mountains, experience new cuisines, meet interesting people from around the world, train with the Shaolin monks, learn urban survival from navy seals, and continually train to become the best version of myself possible and pursue causes that mattered to me. I guess everyone *is* different.

Food and Health

I'm obsessed with food and nutrition. I love to cook and I love to experience the best food I can find. I believe food is the most potent player in the health and longevity of a human being. I eat a Paleo and Primal style diet that consists of some dairy and no grains. I will have a "cheat" meal or two on the weekends, but for the most part I remain gluten-free. If I'm out of town and the occasion calls for it—like in Chicago for deep-dish pizza—I'll have grains. Other than that, I avoid grains because of their inflammatory effects on the body (and so should you).

If there had to be only one thing that you take away from any of my work it would be <u>the importance of food</u>. You have to start eating real food if you want the best results, and/or to enjoy a long and healthy life. There is no way around it--no hack, tip, trick, or shortcut. Maybe when we invent nanotechnology that is able to reverse aging and cure disease, nutrition won't matter. But we don't have that technology, so until we do, food is the epicenter of human existence.

How to eat well:

Avoid anything processed, refined, synthetic, artificial, etc.
Cook your food at home often so you can control the ingredients.
Buy the highest-quality food in its fresh, raw and as close to its natural state as possible.
Don't eat anything that isn't "real food."

My philosophy

I'm a practicing Stoic. In a nutshell, this means I base my decisions on only what is in my control—like my thoughts, emotions and actions—and I avoid wasting time on things out of my control—like other people, the weather, the past, the future. By taking this pragmatic approach to life, one sees how pointless things like anger, jealously, fear, and worry, actually are. Of course, as with everything, it takes practice. I regularly *catch* myself indulging in negative thoughts even though I've always been an optimist and I'm a consciously practicing Stoic.

I have yet to find a more practical way of living life. This would be my second most potent recommendation for you. Learn about Stoicism and other philosophy. Philosophy has the power to change your life. Here are some resources to help you:

Ryan Holiday Article on Tim Ferris Blog
The Art of Living: The Classical Manual on Virtue, Happiness, and Effectiveness

My health and fitness

I average 8-9% body fat year round. This fluctuates up or down depending if I'm traveling or have been eating out a lot lately. I lift 3-4 days a week and target each main lift at least once—squat, deadlift, bench, press. I like to use gymnastics as "accessories" to the main lifts. I practice handstands and the basic holds/moves you see break dancers do (and no, I'm not a breaker... maybe one day). I incorporate some full-body functional training like sled work, farmer carries, and tire flips, at least once a week. I need to remind myself to sprint at least once a week. I just started swimming and am kicking myself for not utilizing this amazing form of exercise sooner.

Life

I'm passionate about life and aim to live each day to the fullest. Although this is tough as I often run into the problem of feeling like I'm not doing enough. This is a fault I struggle with. It's the byproduct of being too forward-minded. I tend to forget what *I've already done* and find myself focusing too much on *what I need to do*. I often have to remind myself to take breaks and spend time with friends and family.

I believe that relationships should be a constant pursuit in our lives. They are one of the most important things, if not thee most important. Unfortunately, I feel like so many of us let our relationships suffer when other things start monopolizing our time. And I think it's a grave mistake. Your work, school, project, or whatever should never take precedence over your relationships. Your relationships should always come first. (This is as much a reminder for myself as it is my advice to you.)

My Work

Nowadays, I work with a couple clients in a consulting capacity to help them improve their web presence and marketing. I manage my two businesses and I spend the rest of my time writing, reading and researching topics of interest.

My ultimate dream is to make my full-time income from my writing. Since you are reading this, you have brought me one step closer to that dream. I don't take that lightly.

Thank you so very much.

My other books are available on Amazon: www.GymLifeBooks.com. I put out a ton of free content on my website AGymLife.com and the corresponding newsletter at GymLifeClub.com. If you want to get all the updates and exclusive list-only content, stop by and subscribe.

If you ever have any questions or need any help, please shoot me an email: ismynamecolin@gmail.com.

I'm here to help any way I can. At the very least, feel free to share your comments by dropping me a quick note. It's always awesome to get words of encouragement from you guys that help me stay motivated. Amazon reviews also help (I print them out and put them on my wall)!

Yours in Fitness,

-Colin Stuckert

Training Reference Guide
Get this in a PDF guide by going to
www.GymLifeClub.com

Here is an easy-to-remember template for your average training week:

Lift weights and train conditioning three times a week.
Do something longer-distance at least once a week.
Do at least one maintenance session a week.
Get outdoors and do random stuff at least once a week.
Walk every day.

A Hypothetical Training Week:

Monday: Squats followed by a sled-conditioning workout. 15 minutes of skill work at a moderate pace.
Tuesday: Play a pick-up basketball game. A 20-minute walk after dinner. A few sets of push-ups and stretching at home.
Wednesday: Bench press and upper body accessory work. Row 2500m at a slow-medium pace. Yoga for 15 minutes as a cool-down.
Thursday: Walk on the beach. Relax and smell the roses. This is known as a "rest day."
Friday: Active recovery session and skill work for 1.5 hours in the gym. Legs sore from earlier in week so decide to work upper-body gymnastics (handstands, dips, rings). Ride bike for 20-minutes at a medium pace to speed up recovery.
Saturday: Lifting session of deadlift, Olympic weightlifting work, and GHD sit-ups. Beach volleyball, walk on beach, enjoy a hard-earned cheat meal.
Sunday: Five-mile bike ride at a leisurely pace. Spend two hours prepping food for week. Do 100 push-ups, sit-ups, and squats at home at a slow-medium pace.

The Training Session Format:

1) Body Temp Warm-up: Jog, Row, and move for 5 minutes until you break a sweat.

2) Dynamic Warm-up: Do movement based exercises at slow/light intensity to warm-up and loosen your joints.

3) Strength: Perform one or two main lifts a day to failure. Follow a program or stick with 5 sets of 5 at a weight you can barely complete on your last set.

4) Accessory Exercises: Choose 2-5 complimentary exercises and perform 8-15 reps over 3-5 sets. For example, do pistols (single-leg squats), weighted lunges, and glute-ham raises on your squat days, and do dips, floor presses and clapping push-ups on your chest/shoulder day.

5) Conditioning: Complete 5-25 minutes of high-intensity conditioning work.

6) Cool-down: Stretch, jog, walk, and keep moving for 5 minutes to let your body cool down gradually.

Set Schemes:
10 sets of 2 reps
8 sets of 4 reps
6 sets of 3 reps
5 sets of 5 reps
3 sets of 10
2 sets of 15+
1 set of 21+

WOD types:
AMRAP (as many rounds or reps as possible in X time) 5, 7, 9, 10, 12, 15, 20+ minutes
For Time: 2,3,4, 5+ rounds of 2, 3, 4, 5+ exercises for X reps (example= 5 rounds of 10 pull-ups, 10 pushups)
For Time: 100 reps of X
Tabata interval: any exercise or combination of exercises (4 min interval = 20 seconds work, 10 seconds rest until 4 minutes is complete)
10 50m sprints with rest between

In a pinch workouts:
Do a home/travel workout

1 mile run
5x 100m sprints
10x 50m sprints
For time: 100 pushups, 100 sit-ups, 100 air squats
For time: 50 push-ups, 50 air squats
For time: 100 burps (or as many as possible in 7 minutes)

Body Temp warm-up (3-5 minutes of light activity):
Row 500m
Run 500m
5 minutes jump rope
Incline walks
Bike

Dynamic Stretching Warm-up (5-7 minutes of movement-based stretching and moving)(mix these up in various reps and sets):
Squats
Lunges
Arm slaps
Arm circles
Wrist rolls
Neck rolls
Side bends
Runner's lunge
Push-ups
Sit-ups
Jumping jacks

Big Lifts for Strength (choose 1-2 for day):
Back Squat and variants: Front Squat, Overhead Squat, Box Squat
Deadlift and variants: sumo, stiff leg, Romanian,
Press and variants: push press, jerk, split jerk, seated
Bench Press and variants: floor press, DB press, incline, decline
Clean and variants: squat, power
Snatch and variants: squat, power

Common accessory exercises (choose 2-4 per strength exercise above as a compliment):
Squats
Deadlifts
Press
Jerk
Push-ups
Dips
Pull-ups
GHD sit-ups
Back extensions
Good mornings
Clean
Snatches
Kettle bell swings

Conditioning (5-20 minutes of various conditioning modalities):
5 mins - 10 mins - 12 mins - 15 mins - 20 mins - 30 mins - 60 minutes (sometimes)
Strongman
Circuits
Intervals (Tabata)
Swimming
Biking
Hiking
Play a sport

Cool-down (move for 3-5 minutes after workout):
Walking
Stretching
Skill work

Resources:
TK links
Travel WODs: Travel WODs sheet
5/3/1 by Jim Wendler
Starting Strength by Mark Rippetoe

GymnasitcsWOD.com
Home workouts: Trainingbox.tv
MobilityWOD.com

Home/Travel WOD workouts requiring no equipment:

-For Time: 10 rounds of: 10 push-ups, 10 sit-ups, 10 squats
-For Time: 50 squats, 50 push-ups, 50 sit-ups
-For Time: 5 rounds of: Run 50m, 10 push-ups
-As many rounds as possible in 10 minutes of: 7 squats, 7 push-ups, 15 sit-ups
-Tabata squats - do as many squats as you can for 20 seconds, rest for 10. Repeat for 4 minutes
-For time: Run 1 mile, 100 Pull-ups, 200 Push-ups, 300 Squats, Run 1 mile
-4x 400M sprints - rest between
-10x 50m Sprint
-Run 1/2 mile 50 air squats – 3 rounds.
-10-9-8-7-6-5-4-3-2-1 sets of sit-ups and a 100 meter sprint between each set.
-Three rounds of: Run 800 meters, 50 Supermans, 50 Sit-ups
-10 push-ups, 10 sit ups, 10 squats – 10x rounds
-200 air squats for time
-3 rounds for time of: Sprint 200m, 25 push-ups
-Run 1 mile, lunging 30 steps every 1 minute.
-Handstand 30-60 second hold on wall and 20 air squats, 5 rounds.
-100 air squats for time
-100 burpees for time
-50 burpees for time
-For time: 4 rounds of: 10 broad jumps, 10 push ups, 10 sit ups
-10 air squats every 1 minute of your 1 mile run
-Run 1 mile for time

The Gym Life List of Usefulness

My Books: www.GymLifeBooks.com

My full library (and more coming soon) of books to help smart people like you get to where you want to be.

The Blog: www.aGymLife.com

I write about fitness, lifestyle, mindset, nutrition and health. New articles go up about once a week and I send an exclusive "only to my list" piece every Sunday.

Join the Gym Life List: www.GymLifeClub.com

The Gym Life Videos: www.GymLifeVideo.com

I make videos when I can find the time. There are a bunch of 20 Second Recipes videos. Check em out.

My Favorite Products: http://agymlife.com/favorite-products/

Living a healthy lifestyle entails utilizing certain tools, supplements, equipment and so on. This is a list of almost all the products I use in my life. All are tested and proven and are produced by reputable companies.

The Gym Life Podcast: iTunes

This is my new big project. Make sure you subscribe for all the updates. There are currently 14 episodes up. Feel free to listen and leave a review!

The Gym Life Library of Useful Stuff: http://agymlife.com/better/

This is a collection of bits of content ranging from books I recommend, quotes, tips, tricks, articles, videos, and anything else I find that I think is useful.

Disclaimer:

Consult a doctor before you engage in any exercise program.

The information provided in this book is designed to provide helpful information on the subjects discussed. This book is not meant to be used, nor should it be used, to diagnose or treat any medical condition. For diagnosis or treatment of any medical problem, consult your own physician. The publisher and author are not responsible for any specific health or allergy needs that may require medical supervision and are not liable for any damages or negative consequences from any treatment, action, application or preparation, to any person reading or following the information in this book. References are provided for informational purposes only and do not constitute endorsement of any websites or other sources. Readers should be aware that the websites listed in this book may change.

This book is designed to provide information and motivation to our readers. It is sold with the understanding that the publisher is not engaged to render any type of psychological, legal, or any other kind of professional advice. The content of each article is the sole expression and opinion of its author, and not necessarily that of the publisher. No warranties or guarantees are expressed or implied by the publisher's choice to include any of the content in this volume. Neither the publisher nor the individual author(s) shall be liable for any physical, psychological, emotional, financial, or commercial damages, including, but not limited to, special, incidental, consequential or other damages. Our views and rights are the same: You are responsible for your own choices, actions, and results.